1

INTRODUCTION

Cialis is a medication permitted through the Food and Drug Administration (FDA) regularly used to deal with erectile disorder (ED) and benign prostatic hyperplasia (BPH) in guys. It is taken as an oral pill either as a low-dose every day medicine or as a better-dose "on-demand" medicine.

Cialis is the brand call for tadalafil, a remedy this is extensively utilized to treat ED. Tadalafil is in a category of medicine referred to as phosphodiesterase-5 (PDE5) inhibitors and is available in a generic shape often called customary Cialis. Tadalafil has been on the market for the reason that 2018 and has the equal primary component as Cialis and is commonly simply as effective — the simplest difference is the rate.

Tadalafil (Cialis) is one of the maximum popular erectile dysfunction (ED) drugs. Its main attraction? The drug is available in low-dose versions that can be taken each day. This method you could have sex at any time, instead of wanting to take a tablet from time to time as needed like different ED manufacturers.

The starting dose for daily-use Cialis is 2.5 milligrams (mg). If that does not work, you could boom your every day dose as much as 5 mg. But is this the proper technique for you—or are you better off with conventional ED pills like Viagra, Levitra, or maybe the nondaily model of Cialis? If you are considering Cialis for day by day use, keep in mind these questions after which talk it with your physician?

1. How often do you have intercourse? If it is or greater times per week, a daily pill might be an inexpensive desire, for the

reason that drug continually circulates for your bloodstream.

2. How important is spontaneity? An each day tablet clears the direction for intercourse at any time—if the drug works for you. (Remember, similar to other ED drugs, it may no longer paintings for all people). On the other hand, the 36-hour window offered through the nondaily model of Cialis would possibly provide enough spontaneity.

3. Have facet consequences of your modern ED pill been bothering you? Taking a each day low-dose pill may additionally lessen facet outcomes, though it may lessen effectiveness as nicely. In studies, the most common day by day pill facet effects had been headache, muscle pain, indigestion, and returned pain.

4. How a great deal alcohol do you drink? Men taking Cialis for each day use can enjoy a worrisome drop in blood strain in the event that they drink an excessive amount of.

5. What other medicines do you take? Ask your physician if any medicines or dietary supplements you take may interact with a each day erectile disorder

pill, such as blood pressure tablets, antifungal capsules, and HIV tablets. Also, men taking nitrate medicines are suggested no longer to take any ED drugs.

6. How essential is value? While the producer suggests that a 30-day deliver of every day Cialis should value about similar to eight capsules of 36-hour Cialis a month, there is no way to put in force this. Check your coverage policy and neighborhood pharmacies for rate statistics.

HOW TO USE CIALIS

Read the Patient Information Leaflet furnished through your pharmacist before you start taking tadalafil and on every occasion you get a refill. If you've got any questions, ask your health practitioner or pharmacist. Take this medicinal drug with the aid of mouth, with or without food, as directed by way of your medical doctor. Do now not take tadalafil greater regularly than once day by day. The producer directs to swallow this medication whole. However, many comparable capsules (immediate-release pills) may be cut up/crushed. Follow your health practitioner's instructions on the way to take this remedy. The dosage is based in your medical situation, reaction to treatment, and other medicines you may be taking. Be sure to inform your physician and pharmacist approximately all the goods you operate (together with prescription drugs, nonprescription tablets, and natural merchandise).

To treat the signs and symptoms of BPH, take this remedy as directed by means of your medical doctor, commonly once a day. If you are also taking finasteride with this remedy to deal with signs of BPH, communicate together with your doctor about how lengthy you need to hold taking this medicine. To treat erectile dysfunction-ED, there are 2 ways that tadalafil can be prescribed. Your health practitioner will decide that is the excellent way with a view to take tadalafil. Follow your doctor's instructions exactly because your dosage relies upon on how you take it. The first manner is to take it as needed, generally at least 30 minutes before sexual pastime. Tadalafil's impact on sexual capacity might also last as long as 36 hours.

The second way to treat ED is to take tadalafil regularly, once a day each day. If you are taking it this manner, you can attempt sexual pastime at any time among your doses. If you are taking tadalafil to treat each ED and BPH, take it as directed with the aid of your physician, typically as soon as an afternoon. You can also attempt sexual hobby at any time between your doses. If you're taking tadalafil as soon as day by day for BPH, or for ED, or for each, take it often to get the most gain from it. To assist you do not forget, take it at the identical time every day.

HOW DO YOU'RE TAKING CIALIS

Cialis is to be had as an oral tablet in several dosages, allowing people to take a low-dose pill every day or a more potent dose on-demand earlier than sexual pastime. The each day doses are available in 2.Five- and five-mg tablets. Doctors commonly begin their patients on the two.Five-mg dose, though five mg can be appropriate if wished for more efficacies. A daily dose of 5 mg may be an excessive amount of for a few human beings and result in undesirable side effects.

On-demand doses are to be had in 10- and 20-mg doses. Doctors normally endorse beginning with a ten-mg dose and moving up to 20 mg if a more potent dose is wanted to gain the preferred effects.

A 2016 studyTrusted Source discovered that while low-dose each day use might also have produced a barely weaker impact than the better-dose, on-call for use in a few take a look at individuals, there did not appear to be a primary gain with one technique over the other.

To get the maximum out of Cialis:

1.   With an on-demand dose, take Cialis at least half-hour previous to sexual activity, although understand that it could absorb to two hours to take effect.

2.   Take daily doses at about the same time each day.

3.   Focus on dealing with strain.

4.   Maintain healthful conversation along with your partner.

TREATMENT COMMUNICATIONS

Although certain drug treatments have to now not be used together in any respect, in other cases two distinct medicines may be used collectively even supposing an interplay might occur. In those instances, your doctor may additionally want to change the dose, or different precautions may be vital. When you're taking this medication, it's miles specifically important that your healthcare professional recognize in case you are taking any of the drugs listed below. The following interactions have been selected on the basis in their capacity importance and aren't always all-inclusive.

Using this medicine with any of the subsequent drugs isn't endorsed. Your physician may determine no longer to treat you with this medication or alternate a number of the opposite drugs you take.

1. Amyl Nitrite

2. Boceprevir

3. Erythrityl Tetranitrate

4. Isosorbide Dinitrate

5. Isosorbide Mononitrate

6. Nitroglycerin

7. Pentaerythritol Tetranitrate

8. Propatyl Nitrate

9. Riociguat

10. Telaprevir

11. Vericiguat

Using this medicine with any of the following drugs is typically now not endorsed, but may be required in some cases. If both medicines are prescribed together, your health practitioner may additionally alternate the dose or how regularly you use one or both of the medicines.

1. Alfuzosin

2. Atazanavir

3. Bunazosin

4. Clarithromycin

5. Cobicistat

6. Conivaptan

7. Darunavir

8. Erythromycin

9. Fosamprenavir

10. Idelalisib

11. Indinavir

12. Itraconazole

13. Ketoconazole

14. Lopinavir

15. Moxisylyte

16. Nefazodone

17. Nelfinavir

18. Phenoxybenzamine

19. Phentolamine

20. Posaconazole

21. Prazosin

22. Ritonavir

23. Saquinavir

24. Simeprevir

25. Simvastatin

26. Tamsulosin

27. Telithromycin

28. Terazosin

29. Tipranavir

30. Trimazosin

31. Urapidil

32. Voriconazole

Using this medicine with any of the subsequent medicines may additionally cause an extended danger of certain facet outcomes, but using each capsules can be the first-rate treatment for you. If each drugs are prescribed collectively, your doctor might also exchange the dose or how frequently you use one or each of the drug treatments.

1. Doxazosin

2. Rifampin

3. Silodosin

FURTHER COMMUNICATIONS

Certain medicines should now not be used at or across the time of consuming meals or ingesting sure varieties of food on the grounds that interactions can also occur. Using alcohol or tobacco with positive drug treatments may reason interactions to occur. The following interactions have been decided on on the idea in their capability importance and aren't necessarily all-inclusive.

Using this remedy with any of the subsequent is commonly no longer recommended, however can be unavoidable in a few cases. If used collectively, your physician may additionally trade the dose or how regularly you operate this medication, or provide you with unique instructions approximately the use of food, alcohol, or tobacco.

1. Grapefruit Juice

Using this remedy with any of the subsequent may also cause an accelerated danger of certain side outcomes however can be unavoidable in a few instances. If used collectively, your health practitioner may also change the dose or how frequently you use this medicinal drug, or provide you with unique instructions about using meals, alcohol, or tobacco.

2. Ethanol

Other Medical Problems

The presence of other medical problems might also affect the use of this medication. Make positive you tell your doctor when you have any other medical troubles, especially:

3. Abnormal penis, such as curved penis and birth defects of the penis (eg, angulation, cavernosal fibrosis, or Peyronie's disease) or

4. Leukemia (blood related most cancers) or

5. Multiple myeloma (blood related most cancers) or

6. Sickle-cell anemia (blood ailment)—Use with warning. May increase chance of unwanted facet outcomes (eg, prolonged erection of the penis).

7. Age more than 50 years or

8. Coronary artery sickness or

9. Diabetes or

10. Hyperlipidemia (excessive lipids or fat within the blood) or

11. Hypertension (high blood strain) or

12. Low cup to disc ratio (eye circumstance additionally called "crowded disc") or

13. Smoking—Use with caution. May growth hazard for non–arteritic anterior ischemic optic neuropathy (NAION).

14. Angina (intense chest ache) or

15. Arrhythmia (irregular heartbeat), uncontrolled or

16. Heart attack (within the closing three months) or

17. Heart failure (inside the last 6 months) or

18. Hypertension (excessive blood strain), out of control or

19. Hypotension (low blood strain) or

20. Retinal disorders (eye hassle) or

21. Retinitis pigmentosa (an inherited eye sickness) or

22. Stroke, current history of— should now not be utilized in sufferers with those situations.

23. Bleeding issues or

24. Stomach ulcers—Use should be decided by way of your medical doctor. May boom your danger of bleeding.

25. Heart or blood vessel disease or

26. Pulmonary veno-occlusive sickness or PVOD (a sort of lung ailment)—Use with caution. May make this situation worse.

27. Kidney sickness, slight or slight or

28. Liver ailment, slight or moderate—Use with caution. The results may be multiplied due to slower elimination of the medicine from the body.

29. Non–arteritic anterior ischemic optic neuropathy (NAION, serious eye condition) in one or each eyes, history of—Use with caution. May growth your chance of having NAION once more.

SUITABLE EXERCISE

Use tadalafil precisely as directed via your health practitioner. Do now not use more of it, do not use it more regularly, and do no longer use it for a longer time than your health practitioner ordered. Also, do no longer prevent taking this remedy without checking first together with your doctor.

This medicinal drug comes with an affected person facts leaflet. Read and follow those commands cautiously. Read it again whenever you fill up your prescription in case there is new information. Ask your physician when you have any questions.

You may additionally take this remedy without or with meals.

Swallow the pill whole. Do now not cut up, spoil, chunk, or crush it. When the use of this remedy for erectile disorder, the capability to have sexual hobby may be stepped forward for up to 36 hours after taking the pill.

Use simplest the emblem of this medication that your physician prescribed. Different brands might not paintings the identical way.

DOSING

The dose of this medicine might be extraordinary for distinct sufferers. Follow your medical doctor's orders or the guidelines on the label. The following information consists of handiest the average doses of this medicinal drug. If your dose is unique, do now not trade it until your doctor tells you to accomplish that.

The amount of drugs which you take depends at the strength of the medication. Also, the range of doses you're taking every day, the time allowed among doses, and the period of time you are taking the medication depend upon the scientific problem for which you are using the drugs.

1.　　For oral dosage form (pills):

2.　　For remedy of benign prostatic hyperplasia (every day use):

3.　　Adults—five milligrams (mg) as a unmarried dose, no more than as soon as an afternoon, taken at the equal time each day.

4.　　Children—Use　　　　isn't endorsed.

5.　　For remedy of erectile dysfunction (as wished):

6. Adults—10 milligrams (mg) as a unmarried dose, no more than once a day, taken 30 minutes earlier than you observed sexual activity can also occur. Your medical doctor can also alter your dose as wanted.

7. Children—Use isn't always recommended.

8. For treatment of erectile dysfunction (each day use):

9. Adults—2.5 milligrams (mg) once an afternoon, taken at the equal time each day, with out regard for the timing of sexual activity. Your medical doctor may additionally regulate your dose as wished.

10. Children—Use isn't recommended.

11. For remedy of erectile disorder and benign prostatic hyperplasia (daily use):

12. Adults—5 milligrams (mg) as soon as a day, taken at the same time each day, with out regard for the timing of sexual pastime.

13. Children—Use is not endorsed.

14. For treatment of pulmonary arterial hypertension:

15. Adults—forty milligrams (mg) (two 20 mg pills) taken once a day. Take each drug at the equal time each day. Do not divide the forty mg dose. Your physician can also alter your dose as needed.

16. Children—Use and dose have to be decided by way of your medical doctor.

MISSED DOSE

If you omit a dose of this medicinal drug, take it as quickly as viable. However, if it is almost time for your subsequent dose, bypass the neglected dose and cross lower back for your ordinary dosing time table. Do not double doses.

Store the medication in a closed box at room temperature, away from warmth, moisture, and direct light. Keep from freezing.

Keep out of the reach of youngsters.

Do no longer hold old remedy or remedy now not wanted. Ask your healthcare professional the way you have to get rid of any medication you do no longer use.

SAFETY MEASURES

It is crucial which you tell all your docs which you take tadalafil. If you want emergency medical care for a coronary heart hassle, it is essential that your medical doctor knows while you final took tadalafil.

If you will be taking this remedy for pulmonary arterial high blood pressure, it is very vital that your health practitioner check your development at regular visits. This will permit your health practitioner to peer if the medication is operating properly and to determine in case you should hold to take it. Blood and urine tests can be wanted to test for undesirable effects. If you are taking tadalafil for pulmonary arterial hypertension, do now not take Cialis® or other PDE5 inhibitors, consisting of sildenafil (Revatio® or Viagra®) or vardenafil (Levitra®). Cialis® additionally contains tadalafil. If you are taking too much tadalafil or take it collectively with those medicines, the danger for side outcomes may be better. If you revel in a prolonged erection for extra than 4 hours or a painful erection for greater than 6 hours, touch your medical doctor without delay. This circumstance may additionally require activate clinical treatment to prevent severe and permanent damage to your penis. This medicine does not defend you against sexually transmitted a sickness (which includes HIV or AIDS). Use protecting measures and ask your doctor if you have any questions on this. It is vital to inform your health practitioner approximately any coronary heart problems you've got now or might also have had within the past. This remedy can reason serious facet outcomes in patients with heart problems.

Do not use this medication in case you also are using riociguat or a nitrate medicinal drug, frequently used to deal with angina (chest ache). Nitrate medicines consist of nitroglycerin, isosorbide, Imdur®, Nitro-Bid®, Nitrostat®, Nitro-Dur®, Transderm Nitro®, Nitrol® Ointment, and Nitrolingual® Spray. Some illegal ("road") drugs called "poppers" (inclusive of amyl nitrate, butyl nitrate, or nitrite) additionally incorporate nitrates. If you need to apply a nitrate medicinal drug, take it at least 48 hours after your last dose of tadalafil.

Do no longer drink immoderate amounts of alcohol (eg, five or greater glasses of wine or 5 or greater shots of whiskey) while taking tadalafil. When taken in extra, alcohol can growth your chances of getting a headache or dizziness, growth your heart charge, or lower your blood pressure. If you experience surprising lack of vision in one or both eyes, touch your health practitioner without delay.

Check together with your physician right away when you have a surprising lower in listening to or lack of hearing, which may be observed by means of dizziness and ringing inside the ears. Do now not eat grapefruit or drink grapefruit juice at the same time as you're using this medicine. Grapefruit and grapefruit juice may also exchange the amount of this medication that is absorbed inside the frame. Do not take other medicines except they have been mentioned together with your physician. This consists of prescription or nonprescription (over-the-counter [OTC]) drugs and herbal or nutrition dietary supplements.

SIDE EFFECTS

Along with its needed effects, a medication might also reason a few unwanted effects. Although no longer all of these facet outcomes may occur, in the event that they do occur they may want clinical attention.

Check together with your health practitioner right away if any of the following aspect outcomes occur:

Fewer commonplaces

1. Arm, returned, or jaw pain

2. Blurred vision

3. Chest pain, pain, tightness, or heaviness

4. Chills

5. Cold sweats

6. Confusion

7. Dizziness

8. Fainting

9. Faintness or lightheadedness whilst getting up suddenly from a mendacity or sitting function

10. Rapid or abnormal heartbeat

11. Headache

12. Hearing loss

13. Multiplied erection

14. Nausea

15. Nervousness

16. Ache or discomfort within the arms, jaw, again, or neck

17. Pounding within the ears

18. Sluggish or speedy heartbeat

19. Spontaneous penile erection

20. Sweating

21. Uncommon tiredness or weakness

22. Vomiting

EXTRAORDINARY

Painful or prolonged erection of the penis

Incidence now not regarded

1. Blindness

2. Blistering, peeling, or loosening of the pores and skin

3. Cough

4. Cracks inside the skin

5. Decrease or change in vision

6. Diarrhea

7. Difficulty with speakme

8. Double imaginative and prescient

9. Rapid, abnormal, pounding, or racing heartbeat or pulse

10. Headache, extreme and throbbing

11. Hives or welts, itching, pores and skin rash

12. Incapability to move the fingers, legs, or facial muscle tissues

13. Inability to talk

14. Joint or muscle pain

15. Loss of heat from the body

16. Numbness or tingling of the face, palms, or ft

17. Pink skin lesions, regularly with a pink center

18. Red, indignant eyes

19. Crimson, swollen pores and skin

20. Redness of the skin

21. Redness or pain of the eyes

22. Scaly pores and skin

23. Sluggish speech

24. Sores, ulcers, or white spots in the mouth or on the lips

25. Belly ache

26. Sudden cardiac death

27. Swelling of the ft or lower legs

Some aspect results may additionally arise that commonly do no longer need clinical attention. These side results may work away at some stage in treatment as your body adjusts to the drugs. Also, your health care expert may be capable to tell you approximately ways to prevent or reduce a number of these side results. Check along with your fitness care expert if any of the subsequent side outcomes retain or are bothersome or if you have any questions about them:

More commonplace

1.   Belching

2.   Heartburn

3.   Indigestion

4.   Belly   discomfort, dissatisfied, or ache

LESS NOT EXTRAORDINARY

1.   Bloody nose

2.   Frame aches or pain

3.   Burning, crawling, itching, numbness, prickling, "pins and needles", or tingling emotions

4.   Burning, dry, or itching eyes

5.   Burning feeling in the chest or stomach

6.   Congestion

7.   Trouble with transferring

8.   Trouble with swallowing

9.   Dry mouth

10.   Dryness or pain of the throat

11.   Excessive eye discharge

12.   Eye ache

13.   Feeling of steady motion of self or environment

14.   Feeling of warmth, redness of the face, neck, arms and every now and then, upper chest

15. Fever

16. Hoarseness

17. Lack or lack of power

18. Unfastened stools

19. Muscle aching, cramping, or stiffness

20. Neck ache

21. Ache in the palms or legs

22. Ache or burning inside the throat

23. Redness, pain, swelling of the eye, eyelid, or internal lining of the eyelid

24. Decreased sensitivity to the touch

25. Runny or stuffy nostril

26. Sensation of spinning

27. Sleepiness or unusual drowsiness

28. Stomach disenchanted

29. Swelling of the eyelids

30. Swelling or puffiness of the eyes or face

31. Swollen joints

32. Tearing

33. Gentle, swollen glands inside the neck

34. Tenderness in the belly location

35. Trouble with dozing

36. Higher stomach ache

37. Voice adjustments

38. Watering of the eyes

INFREQUENT

Changes in coloration imaginative and prescient

Other side effects not listed can also occur in some sufferers. If you word any other consequences, check with your healthcare professional.

Call your medical doctor for scientific recommendation approximately facet results. You might also record side consequences to the FDA at 1-800-FDA-1088.

THE END

Printed in Great Britain
by Amazon